South Beach Diet: The South Beach Diet Plan for Beginners

south beach diet cookbook - 70 recipes

Sharon Jackson

The information herein is offered for informational purposes solely, and is universal as so. The presentation of the information is without contract or any type of guarantee assurance.

The trademarks that are used are without any consent, and the publication of the trademark is without permission or backing by the trademark owner. All trademarks and brands within this book are for clarifying purposes only and are the owned by the owners themselves, not affiliated with this document.

Introduction

Thank you for downloading this book, "South Beach Diet - the South Beach Diet Plan for Beginners."

Do you love to eat? If you are a foodie, like me, you will absolutely hate the idea of counting your calories while eating. The constant watching of calories can really take the fun out of eating. If you are someone that keeps track of the current cooking trends, you will know what the South Beach diet is. It's covered in almost every restaurant menu, magazine, newspaper and even TV show. The South Beach diet encourages cooking of a variety of ingredients in a healthy fashion. I promise you that this is not just another low-carb diet. The South Beach program does not fall under the low-carb or low-fat category. In fact, you can enjoy most foods without having to give up on them completely.

This book focuses on almost all aspects of this trendy diet, including the recipes. We wanted to come up with a South Beach diet cookbook which will offer our readers a comprehensive list of recipes. You never want to run out of recipes when on a diet plan. In this guide, we are providing you a plethora of South Beach diet recipes including the South Beach diet food list. We assure you that this 3-phase diet will not only give you the desired weight loss results but it will be fun too. Unlike most other diets that put a lot of restrictions on what you eat, this diet gives you the complete freedom to choose you own carbohydrates and fats. This diet aims at promoting a healthy lifestyle, which will reap permanent benefits to the dieters who use it.

It is our sincere request to follow all the recipes just as they are written. These recipes have been specially created keeping in mind all the needs of this magical diet. Let's get ready to have some fun. Happy reading!

Thanks again for downloading this book, I hope you enjoy it!

Table of Contents

Chapter 1: About the South Beach Diet

South Beach diet is a new way of life, which encourages you to consume the right fats and carbohydrates. Dr. Arthur Agatston developed it in 2003. This diet consists of three phases, where you are not allowed to eat potatoes, rice, baked foods, sugar or fruit in the first phase. Gradually, carbohydrates are added in the second phase, while the third phase focuses on redefining your diet completely, eventually resulting in weight loss. In the first couple of weeks, the carbohydrate consumption is very limited. This means no starchy foods, sugar, fruits or alcohol, although you can gorge on as many eggs as you wish. Sugar-free sweeteners, most cheeses, certain nuts or even coffee can be consumed. As per the diet, this alone can help you lose 2 to 3 kilos in the first couple of weeks.

During the second phase, you can consume fresh fruits, fiber baked foods, whole-wheat pasta, spaghetti and a certain amount of starch. Once you follow the second phase diet, you should be able to shed about half a kilo. Although the weight loss may seem less, the goal is to remain consistent. It is extremely vital that you stick to the diet plan and avoid falling off track.

In the third and final phase, your diet will be completely redefined, preferably for life. The good news is that you can actually eat whatever it is that you want. The South Beach diet does not put any limits on the kind of carbohydrates you wish to consume. However, one needs to remember not to exceed the specified limit. You will need to aim at portion control rather than having to give up on your favorite foods.

Foods that are allowed on South Beach diet

Phase-1 foods -

Meats/Proteins

- Ground beef
- Lean lamb, fat trimmed
- Boiled ham & bacon
- Eggs
- Turkey bacon
- Soy meat substitute

Dairy

- Skimmed or low-fat milk
- Unsweetened yogurt
- Half and half
- Low fat cheeses

Nuts (per serving)

- Around 15 almonds (roasted)
- Around 15 pecans
- Around 15cashews
- 8 roasted macadamia nuts
- 20 peanuts (roasted)
- 3 tablespoons flax seeds

Vegetables and legumes

- Asparagus
- Artichokes
- Green peas
- Celery
- Bok choy
- Leafy greens

- Eggplant
- Mushrooms
- Cucumbers
- Radish
- Rhubarb
- Pickles

Fats
- Oils (olive, canola, corn, grape seed, soybean, sunflower)
- Guacamole (1/2 cup)
- Up to 15 olives
- Margarines

Toppings
- Hot sauce
- Up to 2 tablespoons salsa
- ½ tablespoon steak sauce
- ½ tablespoon soy sauce
- 1 tablespoon Worcestershire sauce

Spices & sweets
- All spices
- All types of extracts
- All types of pepper
- Sugar free cocoa powder
- Gelatin
- Sugar-free popsicles
- Sugar substitutes (stevia, saccharin, sucralose)

Phase 2 Foods

Fruits

- Apples
- All types of berries
- Grapes
- Grapefruit
- Kiwis
- Apricots
- Mango
- Oranges
- Pears
- Peaches

Dairy

- Flavored yogurt

Starches

- Whole-wheat breads
- Whole-wheat bagels
- Whole-wheat pasta
- Whole-wheat spaghetti
- Bran muffins
- Sweet potatoes
- Wild rice
- Brown rice
- Green peas

Vegetables/Legumes

- Barley
- Black-eyed peas
- Pinto beans

Phase 3 foods

- Anything and everything in limited proportions

Chapter 2: Is the South Beach diet a low-carb diet and how is it different from other low-carb diets?

The South Beach diet derives its name from the popular beach of Miami. Most people confuse the South Beach diet as merely a low-carb diet. While it's true that it limits your carbohydrate intake, the South Beach diet is much more than that. This diet does not require you to count your carbs, while encouraging healthy fats and high protein content.

There are several other low-carb diets that are popular at this time, such as the Atkins diet. A lot of people seem to confuse the two but, in reality, they are polar opposites. Even though the structure of these two diets is similar, they operate on different principles. There are several food restrictions on the Atkins diet, which makes it boring to stick to, whereas the South Beach diet only emphasizes on portion control without restricting you from too many foods. Unlike the other low-carb diets, the South Beach diet focuses on "glycemic index" while allowing the dieters the freedom to eat without measuring the calories.

Almost every other diet will require you to watch your calorie intake for every meal, but not the South Beach diet. This is one of the major reasons why the South Beach diet has become increasingly popular in recent years. It encourages the consumption of complex carbohydrates that are rich in fiber such as whole grain breads or brown rice. Dr. Agatston had a completely different approach to the South Beach diet. He said, "It is my purpose to teach neither low-fat nor low-carb. I want you to learn to choose the right fats and the right carbs."

Chapter 3: South Beach diet FAQs

Who can follow the South Beach diet, are there any restrictions?

People who are below 18 years of age or suffering from anorexia, celiac disease, dialysis, hypoglycemia, kidney disease or pregnant ladies are considered to be unsuitable candidates for this diet.

Can I Consume alcohol while on this diet?

Yes, but only during phase 2 and phase 3, that too in limited quantities.

Should I exercise while on this diet?

Most certainly. Exercise will help you lose more weight while on this diet. However, you don't have to do high intensity workouts. 30 minutes of walking or running each day should keep you in the best shape and be sufficient.

I am a vegan; can I still follow this diet?

No, it does not match the needs of the vegan diet.

What if I am allergic to specific foods form the South Beach diet ingredients?

You can consult a South Beach diet counselor in that case.

Can I snack on foods while on this diet?

Yes you can, just remember to stick to the food list if you do so.

Can I follow this diet if I am suffering from diabetes?

Yes, this diet is suitable for diabetes patients. However, we would strongly recommend you to consult your physician before you start this diet plan.

Is the diet high in saturated fats?

The South Beach diet is high in healthy fats while scoring low in saturated fats.

Chapter 4: South Beach Breakfast Recipes

1. Bacon and cheese casserole (Phase 1)

Ingredients

- 1 bunch of kale
- 1 tablespoon olive oil
- 4 bacon slices
- ¾ cup low-fat cheese
- 10 eggs
- ½ teaspoon salt
- ½ teaspoon ground pepper
- 1 teaspoon spike seasoning

Method

- Preheat the oven to 180 degree C.
- Grease a saucepan with some cooking spray and heat it over medium flame.
- Add the bacon slices and cook until browned. Remove and place on a plate. Now add kale leaves in the same saucepan and cook from both sides until crisp.
- IN a casserole dish, layer kale leaves, bacon strips and cheese.
- In a bowl, combine eggs with salt, pepper, spike seasoning and beat well using a fork.
- Pour this batter over the casserole and bake for about 25 minutes until browned.
- Serve hot.

2. Sausage and cheese breakfast cups (phase 1)

Ingredients

- 4 oz turkey sausages
- ½ green bell pepper, chopped
- 1 small onion, finely chopped
- 5 large eggs
- 1 ½ cup sliced button mushrooms
- ½ cup cheddar cheese
- ¼ teaspoon ground black pepper
- ½ teaspoon olive oil

Method

- Preheat the oven to 180 degree C.
- Heat half a teaspoon of olive oil in a large saucepan over a medium flame.
- Add the sausages and cook them until browned from all sides. Add onion and bell peppers, and cook for a couple of minutes.
- Stir in the eggs along with mushrooms and remove from flame.
- Pour into baking molds and bake for 20 minutes. Allow to cool of for 5 more minutes and serve.

3. Turkey patties with fennel (phase 1)

Ingredients

- 1 lb ground turkey
- 1 small onion, minced
- 1 egg, lightly beaten
- 2 tablespoons pecans, finely chopped
- ¼ teaspoon crushed fennel seeds
- ¼ teaspoon salt
- ¼ teaspoon ground black pepper
- ½ teaspoon olive oil

Method

- In a bowl, combine turkey with some chopped onion, pecans, eggs, salt, pepper and fennel seeds and mix well using a spoon. Now, using your hands, make round patties out of this mixture.
- Heat half a teaspoon of olive oil in a large saucepan over a medium flame.
- Place the patties into the pan and cook them for 5 minutes on each side until browned.
- Serve immediately.

4. Tuscan baked eggs and tomatoes

(Phase 1 & 2)

Ingredients

- 1 tablespoon extra virgin olive oil
- 1 small red onion, finely chopped
- 1 teaspoon minced garlic
- 1 cup diced tomatoes
- 1 tablespoon thyme leaves, dried
- 4 medium eggs
- 2 tablespoons grated parmesan cheese
- 1 tablespoon chopped chives
- ¼ teaspoon salt
- ¼ teaspoon ground black pepper

Method

- Heat some olive oil in a large saucepan over a medium flame.
- Add minced garlic, chopped onion and sauté until golden brown.
- Add diced tomatoes and cook until they are completely tender and thickened.
- Add some salt, thyme, chives and mix well with a spoon.
- Pour the mixture into a large casserole dish. Now crack the eggs in the middle of the dish and place the casserole over the flame.
- Cook for 5 to 7 minutes and transfer onto a large plate. Sprinkle on some cheese, ground pepper and serve.

5. Low-carb vanilla ricotta crepes with strawberries (Phase 2)

Ingredients

- 4 tablespoons low-fat ricotta cheese, divided
- ½ teaspoon sweetener + ½ teaspoon for garnish
- 2 eggs
- ½ teaspoon vanilla essence
- 1 teaspoon vegetable oil
- Strawberries, chopped
- 1/8 teaspoon sea salt

Method

- In a bowl, combine the eggs, sweetener, vanilla extract, salt and whisk using a spoon.
- Heat some vegetable oil in a large saucepan over a medium flame.
- Slowly pour the batter over the pan and spread it across the bottom.
- Cook for a couple of minutes until you see a golden crust and flip it over. Cook it for another few minutes and transfer onto a plate.
- Sprinkle 2 tablespoons of ricotta cheese and wrap it.
- Drizzle some more sweetener and chopped strawberries on top and serve. Repeat this for the next crepe.

6. Easy peanut butter oatmeal (Phase 1)

Ingredients

- 1 cup oatmeal
- 1/8 teaspoon sea salt
- ¾ cup water
- 4 tablespoons peanut butter
- 2-3 toasted almonds

Method

- Add some water to a pot, slide in the oatmeal, some salt and stir using a spoon.
- Now cover and cook the oatmeal on medium heat for 4 minutes.
- Remove the lid, add some peanut butter and cook for another couple of minutes.
- Transfer into two separate bowls.
- Using a kitchen knife, chop up the almonds, sprinkle them on top of the oatmeal bowl and serve.

7. Veggie frittata (Phase 1 & 2)

Ingredients

- 1 small red bell pepper
- 1 small zucchini, grated
- 1 small tomato, chopped
- 2 medium eggs, slightly beaten
- ¾ cup skimmed milk
- ¼ teaspoon oregano
- ¼ teaspoon thyme
- ¼ teaspoon sea salt
- 1 tablespoon parsley

Method

- Grease a saucepan with some cooking spray and heat it over a medium flame.
- Add red bell pepper, chopped tomato and zucchini and cook until the ingredients are tender.
- In a bowl, combine eggs with some milk, oregano, thyme, salt, parsley and mix well.
- Stir this mixture into the saucepan and cook on a low flame until the eggs turn firm.
- Transfer onto a large plate and serve.

8. Spanish omelet (Phase 1)

Ingredients

- 1 large egg + 2 large egg whites
- 1/8 teaspoon sea salt
- 1/8 teaspoon ground black pepper
- 1 tablespoon olive oil
- 1 medium scallion, chopped
- 1 small tomato, diced
- 3 olives, sliced
- 1 tablespoon green chili peppers, diced
- 2 tablespoons low-fat cheddar cheese

Method

- In a bowl, combine egg, egg white, ground pepper, sea salt and mix well.
- Heat some olive oil in a large saucepan over a medium flame.
- Slide the egg mixture into the pan and spread it across the bottom. Cook for 30 seconds and then sprinkle some olives, tomatoes, chili peppers and scallions and cover the pan with a lid.
- Cook on a low flame for 5 to 6 minutes and flip it. Cook for another minutes and serve on a large plate.

9. Egg muffins with bell peppers and salami (phase 1 & 2)

Ingredients

- 1 cup salami, diced
- 1 green bell pepper, chopped
- 4 onion greens, finely chopped
- ¼ cup cheddar cheese or Mexican blend cheese
- 10 medium eggs, well beaten

Method

- Preheat the oven to 180 degree C.
- In a bowl, combine the eggs with salami, green bell pepper, onion greens, cheddar cheese and mix well using a spoon or a beater.
- Pour the batter into small silicon molds and set them inside the oven.
- Bake them for 30 minutes until they turn golden brown.
- Serve immediately.

10. Apple cinnamon Crockpot oatmeal (Phase 2 & 3)

Ingredients

- 2 cups rolled oats
- 4 cups water
- 5 cups low-fat milk
- 1 large red apple, skinned and diced
- 1 teaspoon ground cinnamon
- 1 teaspoon vanilla extract
- ½ teaspoon salt

Method

- Grease the bottom of the Crockpot with some oil or butter.
- In a bowl, combine oats, water, milk, apple, cinnamon, and vanilla, salt and mix well.
- Pour this mixture into the Crockpot and cook for 8 hours on low, while stirring it occasionally before you go to bed.
- Remove from flame in the morning and refrigerate for an hour.
- Serve chilled.

11. Quinoa breakfast cake (Phase 1 & 2)

Ingredients

- 6 medium eggs
- 3 cups quinoa, cooked
- 1 cup baby spinach
- ½ cup sliced shitake mushrooms
- ½ teaspoon minced garlic
- ¼ teaspoon sea salt
- ¼ cup shredded cheddar cheese

Method

- Preheat the oven to 180 degree C.
- In a bowl, crack the eggs and beat them lightly using a spoon. To this, add quinoa, spinach, mushrooms, minced garlic, shredded cheese some salt and mix again.
- Pour the mixture into a baking tray and bake for 25 to 30 minutes.
- You can garnish the cake with some fresh cherries on top and serve.

12. Flax seed meal pancakes (Phase 1)

Ingredients

- 1 cup flaxseed meal
- 4 eggs, beaten
- 1/3 cup almond milk
- 1 tablespoon lemon juice
- 1 teaspoon baking soda
- 1 teaspoon vanilla essence
- 1 teaspoon ground cinnamon
- 1/8 teaspoon sea salt
- 2 drops of stevia (optional)

Method

- In a bowl, combine all the ingredients together and whisk lightly using a beater. If the mixture is too thick, add more almond milk.
- Grease a flat saucepan with some butter and heat it over a medium flame.
- Pour the batter over the pan and spread it across the bottom. Cook for 3 minutes until you see bubbles getting formed and then flip it over. Cook for another 3 minutes and transfer onto a plate.
- Serve along with your favorite fruit.

13. South Beach friendly mock French toast (Phase 1)

Ingredients

- 1 cup low-fat ricotta cheese
- 1 large egg
- 1 teaspoon vanilla extract
- 1 teaspoon ground cinnamon
- 2 Splenda packets

Method

- Crack the egg in a large bowl and beat it lightly using a spoon or a beater.
- Now add some shredded cheese, vanilla extract, cinnamon, and Splenda and beat again.
- Grease a flat saucepan with some butter and heat it over a medium flame.
- Pour the batter over the pan and spread it across the bottom. Cook for 3 minutes until you see bubbles getting formed and then flip it over. Cook for another 3 minutes and transfer onto a plate.
- You can add some maple syrup on top if required.

14. Buttermilk waffles (Phase 2 & 3)

Ingredients

- 1 cup whole-wheat flour
- 1 cup rolled oats
- 1 tablespoon baking powder
- 3 tablespoons canola oil
- ¼ teaspoon salt
- 1 large egg
- ½ cup water
- 3 stevia drops
- 1 ¼ cups buttermilk
- ¾ cup sugar-free raspberry jam or any flavor

Method

- In a bowl, combine flour with some oats, baking powder and salt and mix well.
- In another bowl, combine egg, oil, water, buttermilk, Stevia drops and whisk lightly. Now pour the buttermilk mixture into the oats mixture and stir well using a large spoon.
- Grease a flat waffle iron with some butter.
- Pour half the batter over the iron and cook until the waffles are nice and crisp. Repeat the process for the remaining batter.
- Garnish with a dollop of raspberry jam and serve.

15. South Beach friendly ricotta custard (Phase 1)

Ingredients

- ¾ cup low-fat ricotta cheese
- 4 oz low-fat cream cheese
- ½ cup sugar substitute
- 1 large egg + 1 egg white
- ¼ teaspoon vanilla extract
- ½ teaspoon ground cinnamon
- ¼ cup half and half

Method

- Preheat the oven to 220 degree C.
- In a bowl, combine ricotta with cream cheese and beat until nice and creamy.
- Now add some sugar substitute, egg and egg white, vanilla extract, ground cinnamon, half and half and beat it lightly with a beater.
- Pour the batter into ramekins. Pour some hot water into the baking dish and place the ramekins over it.
- Bake for 45 minutes and chill in the refrigerator for an hour before serving.

16. South Beach friendly chocolate milkshake (All phases)

Ingredients

- 2 cups skimmed milk
- 3 tablespoons cocoa powder
- 1 tablespoon vanilla extract
- 2 teaspoons agave nectar
- 8 to 9 ice cubes
- ¼ teaspoon ground cinnamon

Method

- Combine milk, cocoa powder, vanilla extract, agave and cinnamon in a blender and blend until smooth.
- Now add some ice cubes and whisk again until smooth and frothy.
- Pour into tall glasses and serve chilled.

Chapter 5: South Beach Lunch Recipes

1. Lemon couscous chicken (Phase 2)

Ingredients

- 1 cup water
- 1 cup couscous mix
- 1 tablespoon extra virgin olive oil
- 2 cup broccoli florets
- 1 cup chicken cubes, cooked
- 3 tablespoons lemon juice
- ¼ teaspoon lemon rind
- ¼ teaspoon salt
- ¼ teaspoon ground pepper

Method

- Fill a pot with some water and bring it to the boil. Add some oil, salt and broccoli and cook for a minute.
- Now add couscous mix, cooked chicken, lemon juice, rind and some pepper and simmer for 8 minutes.
- Cover and allow it to stand for 5 minutes.
- Serve hot.

2. Roasted beef wrap (Phase 1)

Ingredients

- 1 cup low-fat cream cheese
- 4 tortillas
- ½ red onion, thinly sliced
- 4 to 5 spinach leaves
- 8 oz roasted beef
- Some ketchup for serving

Method

- Using a sharp knife, chop the beef roast into thin slices.
- Place the tortillas on a plate and spread some cream cheese on them using a spoon.
- Layer them with beef slices, spinach and onion and fold them.
- Serve along with some ketchup.

3. Chicken breasts with tarragon cream sauce (Phase 1)

Ingredients

- 4 medium chicken breasts, skinless
- 1 tablespoon butter, melted
- 1 tablespoon olive oil
- ½ cup low-fat cream
- 1 tablespoon Dijon mustard
- 2 teaspoons fresh tarragon
- ¼ teaspoon salt
- ¼ teaspoon ground pepper

Method

- Season the chicken breasts with some olive oil, salt and pepper and brown them on each side in a large saucepan over a medium heat. Transfer the chicken to a large dish and tent with a foil.
- Add some cream to the same saucepan along with some mustard and tarragon. Stir all the ingredients properly and cook for about 5 minutes.
- Pour the sauce over the chicken breasts, drizzle some melted butter on top and serve immediately.

4. Lemon dill chicken recipe (Phase 1)

Ingredients

- 2 tablespoons olive oil
- 2 tablespoons lemon juice
- 2 minced garlic cloves
- 1 teaspoon dill weed
- ½ teaspoon sea salt
- 2 chicken breasts, sliced into halves

Method

- In a bowl, combine some olive oil with lemon juice, minced garlic clove, dill weed and salt and mix well.
- Coat the chicken with the lemon mixture and allow it to sit for 20 minutes.
- Pre heat the broiler to 220 degree C.
- Broil the chicken breasts for about 8 minutes on each side until tender.
- Serve immediately

5. Chicken stuffed peppers (Phase 2 & 3)

Ingredients

- 2 large red bell peppers
- ½ teaspoon salt
- ½ teaspoon ground pepper
- ¾ cup mozzarella cheese
- 4 tablespoons parmesan cheese
- 2 minced garlic cloves
- 1 cup cooked ground chicken
- ¼ cup finely chopped mushrooms
- 1/4 teaspoon thyme
- 1 small onion, minced
- 1 teaspoon vegetable oil

Method

- Pre heat the oven to 180 degree C.
- Slice the bell peppers into halves and place them on a baking dish. Bake them for 8 minutes.
- Heat some oil in a saucepan and add minced garlic and onion to it. Sauté until golden brown. Add chopped mushrooms, thyme, and cook for 3 minutes until tender.
- Add salt and pepper, stir in the mozzarella cheese, cooked chicken and toss well.
- Fill this mixture inside the bell pepper halves and sprinkle some Parmesan cheese on top.
- Bake for another 12 minutes and serve.

6. Mongolian beef (Phase 2)

Ingredients

- ¾ lb beef steak, boneless and cut into 2 inch squares
- 3 tablespoons cornstarch
- 4 tablespoons teriyaki sauce
- 1 tablespoon sherry
- 1 minced garlic clove
- 1 cup water
- 1 teaspoon white wine vinegar
- ½ teaspoon red pepper flakes
- 2 tablespoons canola oil
- 1 cup onions greens, chopped
- 1 large green pepper, sliced into rings

Method

- In a bowl, combine cornstarch, teriyaki sauce, minced garlic and sherry and mix well. Add the beef chunks and marinate for 30 minutes.
- In another bowl, combine water, teriyaki sauce, vinegar, pepper flakes and mix.
- Heat some oil in a saucepan and brown the beef from both sides. Remove from flame.
- In the same pan, add green onions and bell pepper and fry for 4-5 minutes.
- Slide in the beef, teriyaki mixture, veggies and cook until thick.

7. Southwestern ground beef chili (Phase 1)

Ingredients

- 2 ½ lb ground beef
- 1 small chopped onion
- 1 small green bell pepper, chopped
- 2 tablespoons vegetable oil
- Some chopped cilantro
- 4 tablespoons red chili flakes
- 3 tablespoons ground cumin
- 2 tablespoons minced garlic
- ¼ teaspoon cayenne pepper
- ½ teaspoon salt
- ½ teaspoon ground pepper

Method

- In a bowl, combine cayenne pepper, ground black pepper, salt, cumin and chili flakes and mix well. Coat the beef with this mixture and allow it to sit for 20 minutes.
- Heat some oil in a saucepan over medium heat. Add minced garlic, onions and sauté until brown. Add peppers and cook for 4 to 5 minutes until tender.
- Slide in the beef and cook until browned from both sides.
- Serve hot.

8. Sirloin tips with mushroom (Phase 1)

Ingredients

- 3 tablespoons olive oil
- 3 minced garlic cloves
- 1 ½ lb beef sirloin
- 1 ½ cup button mushrooms, chopped
- 1 cup fresh tomatoes, pureed
- ½ teaspoon salt
- ½ teaspoon ground pepper
- ¾ cup red wine

Method

- Using a sharp knife cut the beef into large chunks.
- Heat some olive oil in a pan and add minced garlic. Sauté until brown and add beef.
- Slide in the mushrooms, tomato puree, pepper and salt and red wine and mix well.
- Cook the mixture for about 30 minutes until brown with the lid covered.
- Serve hot.

9. Baked pesto chicken (Phase 1)

Ingredients

- 4 medium chicken breasts
- ½ teaspoon salt
- ½ teaspoon freshly ground black pepper
- ½ cup basil pesto, homemade or store bought
- 2 oz low-fat mozzarella cheese, grated

Method

- Pre heat the oven to 180 degree C.
- Pat the chicken breasts dry using paper towels and trim the excess fat using a sharp knife. Now slice them up into 2-inch chunks and season them with some salt and pepper. Allow them to sit for 30 minutes.
- Grease a baking tray and lay the chicken over it. Spread a generous amount of pesto sauce over the chicken and cover the tray with an aluminum foil.
- Bake for about 30 minutes. Now add some cheese on top and bake for another 5 minutes until the cheese melts.
- Serve immediately.

10. Roasted winter squash and sausage with herbs (Phase 2)

Ingredients

- 2 pounds peeled and cubed squash
- 5 small turkey sausages
- 2 tablespoons olive oil
- ½ teaspoon dried thyme
- ½ teaspoon salt
- ½ teaspoon freshly ground black pepper
- 2 teaspoons mixed herbs of your choice

Method

- Preheat the oven to 200 degree C.
- In a bowl, combine olive oil, salt, ground pepper, dried thyme, mixed herbs and mix well.
- Now add the squash cubes and toss all the ingredients well. Add them to greased baking tray and bake for 5 minutes.
- Heat a saucepan over medium flame and brown the sausages from all sides. Once done, cut them up into slices and add them to the baking dish.
- Bake for another 12 to 15 minutes and serve hot.

11. Barley risotto with spinach and Parmesan cheese (Phase 2)

Ingredients

- 2 teaspoons olive oil
- 1 small onion, finely chopped
- ¾ cup barley
- 1 tablespoon fresh thyme
- ¼ teaspoon salt
- ¼ teaspoon ground black pepper
- 4 cups chicken broth
- 1 cup baby spinach, thawed
- ¼ cup low-fat parmesan cheese, grated

Method

- Heat some olive oil in a saucepan over medium flame.
- Add chopped onion and sauté until golden brown. Now add barley, salt, pepper, thyme and one cup of broth and simmer for 10 to 12 minutes.
- Now stir in the remaining broth along with baby spinach and stir well. Cook for 8 minutes and transfer into a large bowl.
- Garnish with some shredded cheese and serve.

12. Santa Fe steak (Phase 1)

Ingredients

- 2 tablespoons extra virgin olive oil
- 1 large poblano pepper, sliced
- 1 small onion, thinly sliced
- 1 cup water
- 4 minced garlic cloves
- 1 teaspoon ground cumin
- 1 ½ lbs flank steak
- ¼ teaspoon salt
- ¼ teaspoon ground black pepper

Method

- Heat one-tablespoon extra virgin olive oil in a saucepan over a medium flame.
- Add onion and Poblano pepper and cook for 5 minutes of minutes.
- Add some water, salt and pepper and cook for 4 more minutes until water evaporates.
- In a bowl, combine cumin, garlic, and oil and rub it over the steak.
- Grill it for 5 minutes on each side and transfer to a plate.
- Serve along with onion and peppers.

13. Roast turkey with herbs (Phase 1)

Ingredients

- 1 ½ pound turkey
- ½ teaspoon salt
- 1 orange, thinly sliced
- ½ teaspoon cayenne pepper
- 1 tablespoon chopped parsley
- 1 tablespoon crushed thyme leaves
- 3 tablespoons extra virgin olive oil
- 3 tablespoons dry white wine

Method

- Preheat the oven to 220 degree C.
- Using a sharp kitchen knife, make some slits all over the turkey. Tuck orange slices into these slits and season the turkey with some salt and pepper. Combine thyme leaves, parsley, and 1-tablespoon extra virgin olive oil and rub it all over the turkey.
- Bake in the oven for 30 minutes. Remove the turkey and reduce the temperature to 180 degree F. Baste the turkey with the remaining oil and wine and bake again for 30 minutes more.
- Discard orange slices and serve.

14. Pork satay (Phase 1)

Ingredients

- ¼ cup no-sugar peanut butter
- ¼ cup water
- 1 tablespoon rice wine vinegar
- 2 tablespoons soy sauce
- 2 minced garlic cloves
- 1/8 teaspoon red pepper flakes
- 1 ½ pound pork chunks
- ¼ teaspoon salt
- Metal skewers

Method

- Set the oven to broil.
- In a bowl, combine peanut butter with soy sauce, salt, garlic, red pepper flakes, water and vinegar and mix.
- Coat the pork chunks with half of the peanut butter sauce and marinate for 20 minutes.
- Insert the pork chunks onto skewers and broil for about 4 to 5 minutes on each side.
- Serve along with remaining sauce.

15. Big easy shrimp (Phase 1 & 2)

Ingredients

- 2 strips bacon
- 1 medium onion, finely chopped
- 1 celery stalk
- 1 small green bell pepper, chopped
- 1 minced garlic clove
- 1 cup chopped tomatoes
- 1 bay leaf
- ½ teaspoon ground black pepper
- ½ teaspoon sea salt
- 1 teaspoon hot-pepper sauce
- 1 teaspoon Worcestershire sauce
- 1 lb tiger prawns, peeled and deveined
- 1 teaspoon olive oil

Method

- Grease a saucepan with some cooking spray and cook the bacon in it until crisp. Once done, remove on a paper and crumble
- In the same skillet, add some oil and cook onions, bell pepper and celery until tender.
- Slide in the garlic and cook for a minute. Add bay leaf, tomatoes, Worcestershire sauce and hot sauce and simmer for 20 minutes.
- Add bacon, shrimp, salt, pepper and cook for 5 more minutes.
- Serve hot.

16. Five spice salmon (Phase 1)

Ingredients

- 2 teaspoons grated lime peel
- 3 tablespoons lime juice
- 2 teaspoon extra virgin olive oil
- 1 tablespoon minced ginger
- 1 teaspoon five-spice powder
- ½ teaspoon brown sugar
- 1 lb salmon steaks, sliced into 4 pieces
- 6 cups baby spinach
- 2 minced garlic
- ¼ teaspoon sea salt

Method

- In a large bowl, combine lime peel, lime juice, ginger, five-spice powder, salt, brown sugar and one teaspoon oil and mix. Coat the salmon with this mixture and marinate for 30 minutes.
- In a microwave dish, combine spinach with minced garlic and remaining oil and microwave for 2 minutes.
- Brush the grill with some oil and place the salmon over it. Grill it for 4 minutes on each side.
- Transfer the spinach onto a large plate, place the fish over it and serve.

17. Thai grilled beef with string beans

(Phase 1)

Ingredients

- 1 ½ lb beef steak
- 2 teaspoons olive oil
- ½ teaspoon salt
- ½ teaspoon ground black pepper
- ¼ cup lime juice
- 1 tablespoons fish sauce
- ¼ teaspoon Thai red chili paste
- 1 teaspoon cilantro
- ½ cup scallions, sliced
- 1 lb string beans, cooked and drained

Method

- Season the steak with some salt and pepper.
- Grill for 4 minutes on each side and slice it up thinly.
- In a bowl, combine lime juice, fish sauce, red chili paste, scallions and cilantro and mix.
- Transfer the steak onto a plate, place the beans besides it and pour the sauce all over it.
- Serve hot.

18. Roasted eggplant stuffed with beef (Phase 1 & 2)

Ingredients

- 2 large eggplants
- 2 tablespoons extra virgin olive oil
- 1 small onion, chopped
- 1 green bell pepper
- 2 minced garlic cloves
- 1 lb ground beef
- ¼ teaspoon salt
- ¼ teaspoon ground black pepper
- ½ cup tomato sauce
- 1 teaspoon dried oregano
- ½ cup parmesan cheese, shredded

Method

- Preheat the oven to 200 degree C.
- Pierce the eggplants using a fork. Lay them on a baking tray and roast them for 20 minutes. After they cool down, scoop out the pulp and place onto a large plate.
- Heat some oil in a large skillet. Add minced garlic, onion and sauté until golden brown. Add pepper and cook for a minute. Slide in the beef, salt, pepper, tomato sauce and oregano and cook for 15 minutes until the mixture thickens. Stir in some cheese and mix.
- Stuff this mixture into the eggplants and bake for 15 minutes. Serve hot.

19. Crockpot Balsamic and onion pot roast

(All three phases)

Ingredients

- 1 1/2 lbs chuck roast
- 2 tablespoons steak rub
- 2 tablespoons olive oil
- ¼ cup water
- 2 large onions, sliced
- 1 cup beef stock
- ½ cup balsamic vinegar
- ½ cup thick tomato sauce
- ½ teaspoon salt

Method

- Season the steak with some salt and pepper and steak rub.
- Add some oil to the Crockpot over a medium flame and add the steak. Cook both sides until browned. Remove on a plate.
- Add onions to the Crockpot and sauté until golden brown. Add tomato sauce and balsamic vinegar, and cook for 4 minutes.
- Pour the beef stock, steak and water and cover the lid.
- Cook for 5 hours on high flame. Serve hot.

20. Baked cod with tarragon, basil, white wine and rosemary (Phase 1)

Ingredients

- 1 lb fresh cod
- 2 tablespoons melted butter
- 1 minced garlic clove
- 2 tablespoons white wine
- ¼ teaspoon basil
- ½ teaspoon rosemary
- ¼ teaspoon tarragon
- ¼ teaspoon sea salt
- ¼ teaspoon ground black pepper
- 4 lemon slices
- 2 sliced mushrooms
- 2 tablespoons lime juice

Method

- Preheat the oven to 180 degree C.
- Place the fish on a baking tray. Combine butter with minced garlic, wine, rosemary, tarragon, salt, pepper and basil and pour it over the fish.
- Bake for 15 minutes and pull out the tray. Now add the mushrooms, lemon slices and lime juice and bake for another 10 minutes.
- Allow the fish to cool down for another 10 minutes and serve along with some green salad or whole-wheat bread.

Chapter 6: South Beach Dinner Recipes

1. Broccoli chicken Dijon (Phase 1 & 2)

Ingredients

- ½ cup chicken broth
- 1 tablespoon soy sauce
- 4 cup broccoli florets
- 1 minced garlic clove
- 1 tablespoon olive oil
- 1 pound chicken breasts, skinless and boneless
- 2 tablespoons Dijon mustard
- ½ teaspoon salt
- ½ teaspoon ground black pepper

Method

- Heat some olive oil in a large saucepan over medium flame.
- Add minced garlic and sauté until brown. Add broccoli florets and cook until tender. Remove onto a plate.
- Now add the chicken breasts in the same pan and sprinkle some salt over it. Brown them for about 5 minutes on each side.
- Add chicken broth and cook until it reduces.
- Add Dijon mustard, broccoli and soy sauce and cook for 3 to 4 minutes more with the lid covered.
- Season with some ground pepper and serve hot.

2. Mexican jumping beans (Phase 1)

Ingredients

- 1 small onion, finely chopped
- 1 large green pepper, chopped
- 2 minced garlic cloves
- 1 teaspoon olive oil
- 2 cups kidney beans, rinsed
- 1 cup water
- 2 tablespoons red chili powder
- 2 tablespoons low-fat Mexican cheese blend
- ½ teaspoon salt
- ½ teaspoon ground black pepper

Method

- Heat some olive oil in a large saucepan over medium flame.
- Add minced garlic and onion and sauté until brown. Add green pepper and cook for another minute.
- Add beans, salt, pepper, water and red chili powder and mix well with a large spoon. Simmer for 10 minutes until thick.
- Garnish with some cheese and serve along with some brown rice or tortillas.

3. Baked ziti for dinner (Phase 1)

Ingredients

- 8 oz whole-wheat ziti
- 8 oz ground beef
- 1 cup low-fat mozzarella cheese
- ¼ cup fresh parsley, chopped
- 2 cups thick tomato sauce
- 1 teaspoon oregano
- ½ teaspoon dried basil
- ½ teaspoon garlic powder
- 1/4 teaspoon ground black pepper
- 1/4 teaspoon red pepper flakes
- 2 teaspoons parmesan cheese, grated
- 1/8 teaspoon salt

Method

- Cook the ziti as per the directions on the packet.
- In the meanwhile, heat a saucepan over a medium flame and add beef to it. Cook for 5 minutes until brown while stirring it continuously.
- Preheat the oven to 180 degree C.
- In a bowl, combine beef, ziti, mozzarella and parsley and mix. To this, add tomato sauce, salt, red pepper, black pepper, basil, oregano, and garlic powder and mix well.
- Pour this mixture into a greased baking pan. Sprinkle some Parmesan cheese on top and bake for 35 minutes.
- Serve hot.

4. South Beach friendly shrimp scampi (All three phases)

Ingredients

- 2 minced garlic cloves
- ½ cup red wine
- ¼ teaspoon sea salt
- ¼ teaspoon ground black pepper
- ¼ teaspoon red pepper flakes
- 1 tablespoon low-fat butter
- ½ pound shrimp, deveined and tailed

Method

- Pat the shrimp dry using a paper towel. Now season them with some salt and pepper and let them sit for 30 minutes.
- Melt some butter in a saucepan over a medium heat.
- Add garlic and sauté until slightly golden brown. Add wine and red pepper flakes and simmer until thick.
- Slide in the shrimps and cook until pink.
- Serve along with some brown rice.

5. Hamburger minestrone soup (Phase 1)

Ingredients

- 1 lb ground beef
- 1 medium onion, finely chopped
- 1 cup beef broth
- 6 cups water
- 14 oz tomatoes, diced
- 2 cups thinly shredded cabbage
- 1 cup kidney beans
- 1 teaspoon sea salt
- 1/2 teaspoon ground pepper
- 2 minced garlic cloves
- 2 tablespoons Italian seasoning
- Some grated parmesan cheese for garnish (optional)

Method

- Heat a saucepan over a medium flame and add beef to it. Cook for 5 minutes until brown.
- Add minced garlic and onion and cook until tender.
- Now slide in all the remaining ingredients and simmer for 30 to 40 minutes on medium flame.
- Transfer into large bowls, sprinkle some cheese on top and serve hot.

6. Chicken Cacciatore (Phase 2)

Ingredients

- 4 medium chicken breasts
- 1 ½ tablespoons olive oil, divided
- 8 to 10 button mushrooms, sliced
- ¼ cup chicken broth
- 1 small onion, chopped
- 1 small celery stalk, chopped
- 1 small red pepper, chopped
- 2 minced garlic cloves
- 1 cup diced tomatoes
- 1 teaspoon dried oregano
- ¼ teaspoon salt
- ¼ teaspoon ground black pepper

Method

- Season the chicken breasts with generous amounts of salt and pepper.
- Heat a tablespoon of olive oil in a large saucepan over a medium flame. Add the chicken breasts to it and cook for 3 to 4 minutes from each side. Remove onto a plate.
- Add half a tablespoon of olive oil to the same pan along with mushrooms and cook for 4 minutes. Add minced garlic and onion and sauté for a couple of minutes.
- Now add celery, bell pepper, tomatoes and oregano and cook for 3 minutes until tender.
- Pour stock, along with the chicken and simmer for 12 to 14 minutes with the lid covered.
- Serve hot.

7. Curried cauliflower rice with tofu (Phase 1)

Ingredients

- 1 large cauliflower head
- 1 cup tofu, cubed
- 2 teaspoons olive oil
- 1 large onion, diced
- 1 minced garlic clove
- ½ teaspoon curry powder
- ¼ teaspoon salt
- ¼ teaspoon ground black pepper
- ¼ cup onion greens for garnish
- Some chopped cilantro

Method

- Wash the cauliflower thoroughly and add it to a food processor. Blend until you get a coarse, rice-like mixture.
- Heat one-teaspoon olive oil in a saucepan and add the tofu. Cook for 3 minutes until golden brown.
- In the same pan, heat remaining olive oil over medium heat.
- Add minced garlic and onion and sauté until brown. Add curry powder, cauliflower rice, salt, and pepper and toss well.
- Add tofu and cook for 5 minutes.
- Garnish with some onion greens and cilantro and serve hot.

8. Slow cooker Sicilian chicken (Phase 1)

Ingredients

- 1 ½ lbs chicken breasts, skinless and boneless
- 1 large zucchini, cubed
- 14 oz artichoke hearts, quartered
- 1 packet of Sicilian chicken sauce
- ¼ cup low-fat feta cheese
- ¼ teaspoon salt
- ¼ teaspoon ground black pepper

Method

- Trim the excess fat off the chicken breasts and pat them dry using paper towels. Season them with some salt and pepper and set them aside for 30 minutes.
- Place the chicken breasts in a greased Crockpot. Add zucchini and artichokes and mix.
- Pour the sauce on top and cover with the lid.
- Cook on a high flame for 4 hours.
- Transfer onto a large plate, sprinkle some feta cheese on top and serve.

9. Eggplant Parmesan stacks (Phase 1 & 2)

Ingredients

- 1 large egg plant
- 2 tablespoons olive oil
- ½ teaspoon salt
- ½ teaspoon ground black pepper
- 1 cup pasta sauce
- 1 cup low-fat mozzarella cheese, shredded
- Some fresh basil
- 1 packet whole-wheat spaghetti
- Some water for cooking the spaghetti

Method

- Fill a pot with about 2 to 3 cups of water and bring it to a boil. Slide in the spaghetti and cook for 10 to 12 minutes. Drain the excess water and remove onto a large plate.
- Pre heat the oven to 200 degree C.
- Slice the eggplant into ¼ inch slices and pat them dry using a paper towel.
- Lay them on a greased baking tray, brush on some olive oil and bake for 10 minutes on each side. Remove from oven.
- Place the slices on the spaghetti; pour some pasta sauce over the eggplant along with salt, pepper, basil, some cheese on top and set the tray back in the oven.
- Bake for 20 minutes and serve.

10. Sesame beef strips and stir fry veggies (Phase 1)

Ingredients

- ¼ cup soy sauce
- 1 teaspoon brown sugar
- 3 minced garlic cloves
- ¼ teaspoon minced ginger
- 1 tablespoon sesame oil
- 1 lb beef strips
- Around 8 to 10 baby carrots, thinly sliced
- 6 oz snow peas
- 1 bunch green onions, sliced
- 1 tablespoon toasted sesame seeds
- ¼ teaspoon salt

Method

- In a bowl, combine soy sauce with some minced ginger, garlic, sugar and salt and mix well.
- Heat some sesame oil in a saucepan over a medium flame and add the beef strips to it. Cook in batches until browned from all sides. Remove from pan.
- Now add green onions, carrots and snow peas to the pan and cook for 5 minutes until tender.
- Slide in the beef and pour the sauce over it. Cook for a couple of minutes more.
- Transfer onto a large plate, sprinkle some toasted sesame seeds and serve.

11. Quick lemony baked Basa for dinner (Phase 1)

Ingredients

- 4 medium Basa fish fillets
- 1 tablespoon low-fat butter
- 1 tablespoon lemon juice
- ½ teaspoon lemon-pepper seasoning
- ½ teaspoon garlic powder
- ½ teaspoon paprika
- ¼ teaspoon sea salt
- 1 tablespoon green onion
- 1 tablespoon fresh parsley, chopped

Method

- Preheat the oven to 200 degree C.
- Melt some butter in a saucepan and brush it on all sides of the fish fillets.
- In a bowl, combine lemon juice with lemon pepper seasoning, salt and garlic powder and mix well using a spoon.
- Now coat the fish fillets generously with this mixture and allow it to marinate for at least 30 minutes.
- Grease a baking tray and place the fish fillets over it.
- Bake for 10 to 12 minutes.
- Garnish with parsley and green onion and serve.

12. Spicy shrimp and cauliflower grits (Phase 1)

Ingredients

- 1 head of cauliflower
- 1 lb shrimp, deveined and peeled
- 4 tablespoons extra virgin olive oil, divided
- 1 tablespoon Cajun spice
- ½ teaspoon sea salt
- 2 minced garlic cloves
- ½ cup low-fat cheddar cheese, shredded
- 4 bacon slices, crumbled
- ¼ cup green onion
- ¼ teaspoon ground black pepper

Method

- Wash the cauliflower thoroughly and add it to a food processor. Blend until you get a coarse, rice-like mixture.
- In a bowl, add 2 tablespoons extra virgin olive oil, Cajun spice and shrimps and mix well.
- Heat the remaining oil in a large saucepan over medium flame.
- Add minced garlic, onion and sauté until brown.
- Slide in the crumbled bacon, cauliflower rice, cheese, salt and pepper and cook for 5 minutes.
- Add the shrimps and fry for 3 to 4 minutes.
- Garnish with green onion and serve.

13. Monterey Chicken (Phase 1)

Ingredients

- 4 medium chicken breasts, skinless and boneless
- 1 cup barbecue sauce
- 4 cooked bacon slices, crumbled
- ½ cup Monterey jack cheese or any low-fat cheese of your type
- ½ cup green onion, thinly sliced
- 4 large tomatoes, sliced
- ½ teaspoon sea salt
- ½ teaspoon ground black pepper

Method

- Preheat the oven to 180 degree C.
- Pat the chicken breasts dry using paper towels. Season them with generous amounts of salt and pepper.
- Place the chicken on a greased baking dish. Layer it with bacon, tomato slices, and some cheese and pour some barbecue sauce on top.
- Bake for 30 minutes.
- Garnish with some onion greens and serve.

14. South Beach teriyaki tuna (Phase 2 & 3)

Ingredients

- ¼ cup soy sauce
- 3 tablespoons dry sherry
- 1 tablespoons minced ginger
- 5 oz 4 pieces of tuna steak
- ¼ teaspoon salt
- ¼ teaspoon ground black pepper
- Some stir fried veggies to go along with it

Method

- Clean the tuna properly and pat them dry using paper towels. Now season them with generous amounts of salt and pepper.
- In a bowl, combine soy sauce with minced ginger and dry sherry and mix well. Dip the tuna pieces into this mixture and coat them well. Now refrigerate them for 30 minutes.
- Bring the tuna to room temperature before you start cooking.
- Brush the grill with some cooking oil.
- Place the tuna on it and grill for 5 minutes on each side until you see a nice golden layer.
- Transfer onto a large plate and serve along with some stir-fry veggies.

15. Yummy meat loaf (Phase 1 & 2)

Ingredients

- 1 can thick tomato paste
- ½ cup dry red wine
- ½ cup water
- 1 minced garlic clove
- ½ teaspoon dried basil
- ¼ teaspoon dried oregano
- ¼ teaspoon sea salt
- 1 pound ground turkey
- 1 cup oatmeal
- ¼ cup zucchini, shredded
- 1 egg

Method

- Pre heat the oven to 180 degree C.
- In a bowl, combine red wine with water, minced garlic, oregano and basil tomato paste and mix.
- Add it to a saucepan and bring it to a boil. Simmer for 15 minutes until thick.
- In another bowl, combine ground turkey with zucchini, oatmeal, salt and egg and form a dough using your hands.
- Place it onto a greased baking tray and bake for 45 minutes.
- Pour the tomato sauce on top and bake for another 15 minutes.
- Serve hot.

16. Grilled mahi mahi with Korean sauce (Phase 1)

Ingredients

- 2 large pieces mahi mahi
- ¼ cup soy sauce
- 1 ½ tablespoons rice wine vinegar
- 1 tablespoon sesame oil
- 2 tablespoons stevia
- 1 green onion, sliced
- 1 teaspoon minced garlic
- ½ teaspoon cayenne pepper
- ½ teaspoon sea salt
- 1 teaspoon hot sauce

Method

- In a bowl, combine soy sauce with rice wine vinegar, sesame oil, salt, pepper, Stevia, minced garlic, hot sauce and green onion and mix well.
- Add half of this mixture to a large Ziploc bag along with the mahi mahi and shake well. Marinate for 20 minutes.
- Brush the grill with cooking oil and place the mahi mahi fillets on it. Grill for 3 to 4 minutes on each side.
- Serve along with the remaining sauce.

17. Blackened chicken with agave
(Phase 2)

Ingredients

- 4 medium chicken breasts, skinless and boneless
- 4 teaspoons agave
- 1 tablespoon olive oil
- For the Cajun spice blend
- 2 teaspoons paprika
- ½ teaspoon sea salt
- 1 teaspoon cayenne pepper
- 1 teaspoon ground cumin
- 1 teaspoon thyme
- ½ teaspoon ground white pepper
- ½ teaspoon onion powder

Method

- Preheat the oven to 180 degree C.
- Trim the excess fat off the chicken breasts and pat it with some agave on all sides.
- In a bowl, combine all the ingredients for the spice mix and toss well. Coat the chicken with this spice mixture.
- Sear the chicken from both sides on a saucepan over medium heat.
- Add the chicken to a baking tray and bake for 30 minutes.
- Slice up and serve.

18. Gluten free chicken bruschetta (Phase 1)

Ingredients

- 6 medium roma tomatoes, diced
- 2 minced garlic cloves
- 1 tablespoon olive oil
- 1 teaspoon balsamic vinegar
- ¼ cup fresh basil leaves
- ¼ teaspoon salt
- ¼ teaspoon ground black pepper
- 4 medium chicken breasts
- 2 tablespoons feta cheese, crumbled

Method

- Trim the excess fat off the chicken breasts and pat them dry with a paper towel. Season them generously with salt and pepper and marinate for 20 minutes.
- Brush the grill with some cooking oil and place the chicken breasts over it. Grill them for 4 minutes on each side.
- In a bowl, combine diced tomatoes, basil, garlic, vinegar and oil and mix well.
- Place the chicken in a microwave dish and add the above mixture on top.
- Sprinkle some cheese and microwave for 7 to 8, minutes and serve.

19. South Beach pork and pepper stew (Phase 1)

Ingredients

- 16 oz pork loin
- 2 tablespoons olive oil
- 1 medium green pepper, chopped
- 1 large scallion, chopped
- 2 minced garlic cloves
- 2 cups chicken broth
- Some fresh cilantro
- ½ teaspoon ground coriander
- 2 tablespoons lime juice
- 1 oz Monterey jack cheese
- 3/4 cup white beans, soaked
- 1 jalapeno pepper, sliced
- ¾ teaspoon salt

Method

- Heat one tablespoon of olive oil in a saucepan over medium heat. Add the pork loin and brown each side. Remove from the pan and cut it into slices.
- Add the remaining olive oil to the pan and add minced garlic and scallion. Sauté until golden brown. Add green pepper and cook for another two minutes.
- Add some chicken broth, salt, jalapeno pepper, ground coriander, lime juice and beans and stir all the ingredients.
- Slide in the sliced pork and cook for 20 to 25 minutes until the pork is tender.
- Garnish with some cilantro, jack cheese and serve hot.

20. Stir fry chicken and veggies (phase 2 & 3)

Ingredients

- 3 tablespoons canola oil
- ½ pound chicken breasts, skinless
- 3 cups mixed veggies (mushrooms, broccoli, green beans, asparagus, red bell peppers and scallions)
- 2 tablespoons water
- 2 tablespoons soy sauce
- ¼ teaspoon salt
- ¼ teaspoon ground pepper
- 1 cup baby spinach

Method

- Heat 1-tablespoon oil in a saucepan over medium heat. Add the chicken breasts and cook until browned on each side. Remove from pan.
- Now add the remaining oil to the pan and add all the veggies. Sprinkle some salt, water, baby spinach and soy sauce and fry for 4 minutes on high heat. Add the chicken and cook for another 2 minutes.
- Transfer onto a plate, sprinkle some ground pepper and serve.

21.Two Bean Chili Con Carne (Phase 2)

Ingredients

- 1 tablespoon olive oil
- 1 pound ground beef
- 2 tablespoons chili powder
- ¼ teaspoon cayenne pepper
- 1 green bell pepper, sliced
- 1 small onion, diced
- 4 minced garlic cloves
- 1 teaspoon dried oregano
- 1 tablespoons thick tomato paste
- 2 large cups tomatoes, diced
- 12 oz black beans
- 12 oz pinto beans
- ½ cup tomato sauce
- 1 teaspoon salt

Method

- Heat a saucepan over medium flame and add beef to it. Sprinkle some salt, chili powder and cayenne pepper and cook for about 5 minutes on all sides. Remove onto a plate.
- Add minced garlic, onion, green pepper and oregano to the saucepan and sauté for 3 to 4 minutes until tender.
- Slide in the tomatoes, pinto beans, black beans, tomato sauce and tomato paste and simmer for 12 minutes with the lid covered.
- Add the beef and cook for another 5 minutes.
- Serve hot.

22. Buttermilk and salmon chowder (Phase 1)

Ingredients

- 1 turnip, cubed
- 1 medium onion, chopped
- 1 celery rib, chopped
- 1 bay leaf
- 1 teaspoon dried dill
- 2 cups vegetable broth
- 1 cup buttermilk
- 1 bay leaf
- 12 oz salmon, drained
- 1 cup no-fat yogurt
- 1 tablespoons margarine
- ½ teaspoon salt
- ¼ teaspoon ground pepper
- 1 tablespoon hot sauce

Method

- Combine the turnips, onion, salt, celery, bay leaf, dill, and vegetable broth and add it to a saucepan.
- Bring it to a boil and simmer for 12 to 14 minutes until veggies tenderize.
- Now stir in buttermilk, salmon, yogurt, and hot sauce and ground pepper and cook for 5 to 6 minutes.
- Discard bay leaf and serve.

Chapter 7: South Beach Desserts

1.Red and green fruit salad (Phase 2)

Ingredients

- 1 cup green grapes
- 6 oz raspberries
- 2 Kiwi, peeled and sliced
- 6 oz vanilla flavored yogurt
- 8 oz no-fat Greek yogurt
- 1 tablespoon agave
- ½ teaspoon vanilla extract

Method

- Wash the grapes thoroughly under running water and pat them dry with paper towels.
- In a large bowl, combine the grapes with sliced kiwi, raspberries and mix.
- In another bowl, combine the Greek yogurt with vanilla yogurt, agave and vanilla extract and mix well.
- Add this mixture to the fruit mix and toss all the ingredients well.
- Refrigerate this salad for a couple of hours and serve.

2. Whole-wheat molasses and almond cookies (Phase 2 & 3)

Ingredients

- 6 tablespoons low-fat butter or margarine
- 4 tablespoons stevia
- ½ cup whole-wheat flour
- ½ cup whole wheat pastry flour
- ½ cup almond flour
- 1 teaspoon baking soda
- ½ teaspoon salt
- ½ teaspoon ground cinnamon
- ¼ teaspoon all spice powder
- ½ teaspoon ground ginger
- 1/3 cup molasses

Method

- In a bowl, add the margarine and beat it with a hand beater until nice and creamy.
- In another bowl, combine pastry flour with whole-wheat flour, cinnamon, ginger, spice powder, baking soda, salt and almond flour and mix using a spoon. Add molasses, stir in the margarine and beat again.
- Refrigerate this mixture for 60 minutes and then roll it out using a rolling pin. Cut cookie shaped circles and place them on a baking tray.
- Preheat the oven to 180 degree C.
- Bake for 15 minutes and allow it to cool for 30 minutes before serving.

3. Silken chocolate pudding (Phase 2)

Ingredients

- 16 oz tofu, drained
- 2 tablespoons cocoa powder
- ¼ cup sugar substitute
- 1 teaspoon vanilla extract
- ¼ teaspoon sea salt
- 4 tablespoons low-fat whipped topping
- 2 tablespoons roasted and chopped almonds

Method

- Crumble the tofu using your hands and add it to a bowl.
- To this bowl, add cocoa powder, sugar substitute, salt and vanilla extract and mix. Add this mixture to a blender and blend it until smooth.
- Transfer the pudding into attractive bowls and add a dollop of whipped cream and chopped almonds on top.
- Refrigerate for a couple of hours and serve.

4. South Beach chia chocolate and coconut pudding (Phase 1)

Ingredients

- 1 cup coconut milk, light
- ½ cup water
- 2 tablespoons chia seeds
- 1 tablespoon cocoa powder
- ¼ teaspoon ground cinnamon
- 1 teaspoon vanilla extract
- 1 tablespoon splenda
- Some raspberries for garnish

Method

- Combine coconut milk, water, chia seeds, cocoa powder, cinnamon, vanilla extract and Splenda and add it to a large jar with a lid. Now shake all the ingredients well.
- Refrigerate this mixture for at least a couple of hours or add some ice cubes.
- Garnish with some raspberries and serve chilled.

5. Almond meal Clementine (Phase 1 & 2)

Ingredients

- 5 small sized clementines
- 6 large eggs
- 1 cup sugar substitute (preferably Splenda)
- 2 cups almond flour
- 1 teaspoon baking powder
- ¼ teaspoon salt
- Some water for cooking clementines

Method

- Fill a pot with about 2 cups of water and bring it to a boil. Slide in the Splenda and cook for 45 minutes. Once they cool down, add them to a blender and blend until smooth.
- In a bowl, crack the eggs and beat them lightly. Stir in the almond flour, salt and baking powder, and beat again.
- Add clementine to this mixture and toss.
- Preheat the oven to 180 degree C.
- Pour the batter into a baking tray and bake for 45 minutes.
- Wait for another 15 minutes and serve.

6. Cottage cheese pots de crème (Phase 1)

Ingredients

- 1 cup low-fat cottage cheese
- 3 large eggs
- ¾ cup heavy cream
- ¾ cup water
- ½ cup splenda
- 1 tablespoon vanilla extract
- Some raspberries for garnish

Method

- Preheat the oven to 180 degree C.
- Add the cottage cheese to a blender and blend it until smooth.
- Now add the rest of the ingredients to the blender and give it a whisk.
- Pour the batter into small ramekins. Fill the baking tray with some hot water and place the ramekins on the tray.
- Bake for 35 minutes. Garnish with raspberries and serve.

7. Sweet potato muffins (Phase 2)

Ingredients

- 1 cup almond flour
- 10 large dates, soaked
- 1 cup cooked and smashed sweet potato
- 1 cup vanilla flavored protein powder
- 1 teaspoon ground cinnamon
- 1 teaspoon vanilla extract
- ¼ teaspoon baking soda
- 1/8 teaspoon salt
- 2 tablespoons chopped pecans
- 3 large eggs

Method

- Preheat the oven to 180 degree C.
- Add the soaked dates to a food processor and blend until smooth. Add the puree to a large bowl.
- Now add the remaining ingredients to this bowl except the pecans and beat them lightly. If the batter is too thick, add some milk.
- Pour the batter into muffin molds, top them up with pecans and bake for 20 minutes.
- Allow it to cool for 15 minutes before serving.

8. South Beach friendly pistachio pudding (Phase 1)

Ingredients

- 2 oz ricotta cheese
- 2 tablespoons coconut milk
- 1 teaspoon vanilla extract
- 1 teaspoon almond extract
- 1 packet zero calories stevia
- About 20 pistachio nuts, shelled
- Some sliced pistachios for garnish

Method

- In a bowl, combine ricotta with coconut milk, vanilla extract, almond extract and Stevia and mix well using a spoon. You can also use a hand beater to mix the ingredients.
- Crush the pistachios with a rolling pin and add them to the mixture.
- Refrigerate for an hour.
- Garnish with some more pistachios on top and serve chilled.

9. South Beach sugar-free raspberry yogurt pie (Phase 1)

Ingredients

- 16 oz fat-free yogurt
- 1 packet (4 serving) no-sugar raspberry jello
- ½ teaspoon vanilla extract
- 4 tablespoons non-fat whipped cream

Method

- In a bowl, add the yogurt and jello powder, and beat it lightly using a hand beater.
- Now add this mixture to a microwave bowl and microwave for a minute on high.
- Add some vanilla extract to this mixture and mix well.
- Microwave again for 3 minutes.
- Refrigerate this mixture for 3 hours until it is set.
- Garnish with some whipped cream and serve chilled.

10. South Beach diet cheesecake (Phase 1)

Ingredients

- 8 oz low-fat cream cheese
- 3 large eggs
- 1 cup Splenda
- 1 teaspoon vanilla extract
- For the topping
- ½ cup low-fat sour cream
- ¼ cup splenda
- 1 teaspoon vanilla

Method

- Preheat the oven to 180 degree C.
- In a bowl, combine all the ingredients for the cheesecake and beat them until smooth using a hand beater.
- Pour the batter into a greased baking pan.
- Bake for 35 minutes and allow it to cool down for 15 minutes.
- In a bowl, combine all the ingredients for the topping and spread it over the cheesecake. Bake for 10 more minutes and serve.

11. Crustless cheesecake with sour cream topping (Phase 1)

Ingredients

- 1 lb low-fat cream cheese
- ½ cup Splenda
- ¼ teaspoon almond extract
- 3 medium eggs
- For the topping
- 1 cup no-fat sour cream
- 1/8 cup splenda
- 1 teaspoon vanilla extract

Method

- Preheat the oven to 150 degree C.
- In a bowl, combine cream cheese with Splenda and almond extract and beat it until fluffy.
- Stir in the eggs and beat at a low speed until nice and fluffy.
- Pour the batter in a cake pan. Fill the baking tray with some water and place the cake pan on it. Bake for 20 minutes
- In a bowl, combine all the ingredients for the topping and whisk well. Spread them on top of the cheesecake.
- Refrigerate for 3 to 4 hours and serve.

12. No-bake cherry cheesecake (Phase 3)

Ingredients

- 12 oz cream cheese
- 3 tablespoons splenda
- 1 teaspoon vanilla extract
- 1 cup low-fat cream
- 1 cup pie filling, without sugar
- Some fresh cherries, deseeded

Method

- In a bowl, add the cream and beat it until soft peaks are formed.
- In another bowl, combine cream cheese with vanilla extract and Splenda and beat it with an electric mixer. Slide in the whipped cream and mix well using a spoon.
- Transfer this mixture to small ramekins. Top them up with pie filling, fresh cherries and refrigerate for 3 to 4 hours.
- Serve chilled.

13. Pumpkin cheesecake (Phase 1)

Ingredients

- 15 oz mashed pumpkin
- 1 cup low-fat milk
- 1 cup splenda
- ¼ teaspoon salt
- 3 tablespoons pumpkin pie spice
- 2 large eggs
- 8 oz fat-free cream cheese

Method

- Preheat the oven to 180 degree C.
- In a bowl, combine mashed pumpkin with some salt, Splenda, pie spice and cream cheese and beat with a beater until smooth.
- Crack the eggs into the bowl and beat it once again until nice and creamy.
- Pour the batter into small ramekins.
- Pour the batter into small ramekins. Fill the baking tray with some hot water and place the ramekins on the tray.
- Bake for 35 minutes and refrigerate for 3 hours before serving.

14. Yummy orange almond ricotta cheesecake (Phase 1)

Ingredients

For the crust

- 1 1/2 cups graham cracker crumbs
- 2 tablespoons Splenda
- 4 oz fat-free butter or margarine
- 1/4 cup finely chopped almonds

For the filling

- 1 lb low-fat ricotta
- 2 large eggs
- ¼ cup Splenda
- 1 tablespoon whole-wheat flour
- 1 teaspoon almond extract
- Zest of one orange
- 1/8 teaspoon salt

Method

- Preheat the oven to 180 degree C.
- In a bowl, combine the chopped almonds with Graham cracker crumbs, Splenda and butter and mix well using your hands.
- Grease a cake pan and fill the bottom with the crust filling. Spread it evenly using a spoon. Now bake in the oven for about 12 minutes until golden.
- Combine all the ingredients for the filling in a food processor and blend until the mixture is lump free.
- Now pour the batter over the crust and bake for 55 to 60 minutes.
- Ensure to allow it to cool for at least 25 minutes before you take it out.
- Refrigerate the cake for 5 to 6 hours and serve chilled.

15. Nutty granola (Phase 1)

Ingredients

- 1 cup walnuts
- 1 cup almonds
- ¼ cup sunflower seeds
- ½ cup pecans
- ½ cup shredded coconut
- ½ cup stevia or Splenda
- 2 tablespoons margarine
- ¼ cup dark cocoa powder
- 1 teaspoon vanilla extract
- 2 teaspoons ground cinnamon
- ¼ teaspoon salt

Method

- Add walnuts, almonds and pecans in a bowl filled with water and soak them for 5 to 6 hours.
- Preheat the oven to 200 degree C.
- Add the nuts to a food processor and blend until coarse.
- Melt some margarine on a saucepan over low heat. Add cocoa powder, vanilla extract, and cinnamon and stir well.
- Pour this mixture over the nuts, add sunflower seeds and mix well.
- Grease a baking tray with some butter. Spread the granola mixture across the bottom of the tray and even it out using a spatula.
- Cover with an aluminum foil and bake for 4 hours.
- Once the granola cools down, slice it up and serve with some cold almond milk.

Conclusion

Thank you once again for purchasing this book. Following a weight loss diet has never been this easy. Most diets make you starve, keep you away from your favorite foods, affect your energy levels and, as if this was not enough, they are extremely boring too. I actually had a lot of fun writing this book as much as you would have enjoyed reading it. Sometimes, we start following a diet plan and run out of recipes to cook. After all, it's not easy finding the time to stick to a particular diet amidst the fast pace of city life. We know how stressful it can get and therefore we wanted to come up with as many recipes as possible. We hope these recipes were easy to understand. We have tried our best to keep the language simple throughout the book.

Do write in to us if you like our book. Your feedback will only motivate us to providing you with better content with every book we produce.

Bon Appetit,

Sharon.